Distribution, publication, and copying in any form are prohibited and subject to damages.

TEN HYPNOSES

Copying, publishing, and sharing with third parties are only permitted with the written consent of the author. Please observe the notes on copyright and usage.

Distribution, publication, and copying in any form are prohibited and subject to damages.

Copying, publishing, and sharing with third parties are only permitted with the written consent of the author. Please observe the notes on copyright and usage.

Distribution, publication, and copying in any form are prohibited and subject to damages.

Ingo Michael Simon

TEN HYPNOSES

36
Driving Anxiety

Copying, publishing, and sharing with third parties are only permitted with the written consent of the author. Please observe the notes on copyright and usage.

Distribution, publication, and copying in any form are prohibited and subject to damages.

© 2024 Ingo Michael Simon
All rights reserved.
Independently published
www.ingosimon.com

Important Notes for Urgent Attention:

The contents of this book are based on the practical experiences of the author with hypnosis applications and psychotherapy in a trance state. Although the author has strived for the utmost care, errors or misunderstandings in the presentation cannot be completely excluded. Therapeutic work with people and the application of hypnosis are solely the responsibility of the hypnotist. It cannot be ruled out that parts of this book may be misunderstood or that the application of a presented procedure may cause an undesirable reaction in the client. The author also assumes no co-responsibility if work with a client is carried out with reference to the statements in this book.

The Author:

Ingo Michael Simon studied psychology and education and is a hypnotherapist with practices in southwestern Germany and Switzerland. With the help of hypnosis-supported psychotherapy, he primarily treats people with persistent psychological conditions. His practice focuses on anxiety disorders, pathological compulsions, and psychosomatic illnesses. His therapeutic offerings mainly include classical and modern hypnosis applications and the dreamland therapy he developed himself.

Copying, publishing, and sharing with third parties are only permitted with the written consent of the author. Please observe the notes on copyright and usage.

Distribution, publication, and copying in any form are prohibited and subject to damages.

INTRODUCTION	6
COPYRIGHT AND USAGE	8
HYPNOSIS 1	10
HYPNOSIS 2	15
HYPNOSIS 3	20
HYPNOSIS 4	25
HYPNOSIS 5	30
HYPNOSIS 6	35
HYPNOSIS 7	39
HYPNOSIS 8	44
HYPNOSIS 9	50
HYPNOSIS 10	56
ALL TITLES IN THE SERIES	61

Copying, publishing, and sharing with third parties are only permitted with the written consent of the author. Please observe the notes on copyright and usage.

Distribution, publication, and copying in any form are prohibited and subject to damages.

Introduction

The series "Ten Hypnoses" is very well known in Germany, Austria, and Switzerland as a collection of texts for therapeutic work and is used by numerous psychotherapeutic practices, doctors, therapists, coaches, and other helping professionals. I am pleased to now be able to offer these texts in other countries as well.

Most therapists have their own methods for inducing and deepening trance as well as for exiting trance. Therefore, I have focused on the main part of the hypnosis. The texts in this book can be integrated as the main part into any hypnosis process. The texts in this collection use various hypnosis techniques. I will not explain these in detail, as I assume that users have the appropriate training. It is also not necessary to understand the exact structure or functioning of the different parts. The texts can simply be read aloud, and they will have their effect.

Decide for yourself which text best suits your client or patient at any given time. You can also combine passages from different texts. It is not about using all ten hypnoses in sequence. It is a selection of possibilities.

Copying, publishing, and sharing with third parties are only permitted with the written consent of the author. Please observe the notes on copyright and usage.

I want to emphasize that books cannot replace therapy. Psychotherapy or other therapeutic treatments involve much more. A careful diagnosis is the necessary basis for deciding on the use of methods, including whether hypnosis or one of my texts should be used. Even in this case, preparatory discussions, follow-up discussions during the session, and of course, a therapeutic concept for the sequence of sessions and the content approaches are essential parts of therapy. This cannot and should not be achieved with a collection of texts.

In any case, I wish you much success in your work and I am pleased if my text templates can contribute in a small way.

Ingo Michael Simon

Copyright and Usage

Copying, publishing, and sharing with third parties is prohibited and only permitted with the written consent of the author. Please observe the following copyright and usage guidelines.

This work has been carefully crafted and created to the best of the author's knowledge and personal experience. It comprises text templates and application guidelines for professional hypnosis sessions. The author is a licensed psychotherapist with extensive experience in psychotherapy, coaching, and personal training using hypnotic techniques and methods. Nevertheless, the author and the publisher assume no liability for the accuracy of information, instructions, and advice, nor for any typographical errors. The author and publisher accept no responsibility or liability for the application of these texts and recommendations with clients or patients, nor for any potential consequences or unexpected reactions. It is expressly noted that the application of therapeutic and advisory techniques and formulations lies solely and entirely within the responsibility of the practitioner. This also applies to adherence to the boundaries of legally regulated medical and therapeutic practices. The fact that a book containing action proposals is freely available for sale does not imply that its application with clients or patients is permitted for everyone.

Hypnosis 1

You want to finally feel free and relaxed when driving again... ...It is your firm goal to say goodbye to fear, to completely release it... ...It is your clear intention and strong will to end the fear today... ...to end fear and regain freedom... ...Today, more than ever, you are focused on this goal... ...You are more determined than ever before... ...because now is truly the time to let go of fear and associate a new, free feeling with driving a car... ...You can do it... ...You can do it today... ...You can do it right now... ...in this moment... ...It's amazing how well you can now actually strengthen this determination and take a clear step... ...a step of letting go of fear... ...a step into freedom, into a new sense of confidence... ...You are starting now... ...Today is the end of fear... ...Today begins freedom... ...

You have this desire within you to be able to drive a car again with a free and good feeling... ...to let go of fear and then drive with true calmness... ...to let go of everything that hinders or restricts you when driving... ...You've had this desire for a long time, and today it becomes your biggest and most important goal... ...But it goes even further... ...Today, this goal becomes a firm thought... ...a true belief... ...so strong and stable that you cannot help but turn this thought into reality... ...that your body will follow this thought... ...this thought that says... ...I now truly let go of all fear, and in doing so, I gain freedom and calmness when driving... ...This is the decisive thought... ...the all-important thought... ...It now finds its way into your deepest inner self... ...I now truly let go of all fear, and in doing so, I gain freedom and calmness when driving... ...

Your body feeling is also important and can help you... ...because your body feels fear, it also feels relaxation... ...it feels all your emotions... ...because all moods and feelings also show up physically... ...So it is also important to be and remain physically calm, especially when driving... ...because a calm body helps you to stay calm in your feelings... ...Your body also follows your thought because as soon as you think... ...I now truly let go of all fear, and in doing so, I gain freedom and calmness when driving... ...your body enters this beautiful and calm state that you can now feel, and you remain calm and relaxed in your feelings... ...calm and relaxed when getting into a car... ...calm and relaxed when starting to drive... ...calm and relaxed when steering the vehicle... ...calm and relaxed in traffic... ...physically calm and relaxed... ...emotionally calm and relaxed...

Sometimes it's thoughts and fears that make us feel anxious even before we actually feel afraid... ...we then expect fear and imagine it... ...but now you have the freedom thought... ...your thought of letting go of fear and holding on to freedom and calmness... ...Sometimes it's also our feelings that disturb us... ...But upon closer examination, it's not the feelings themselves that scare us, but the judgments and evaluations of our feelings... ...because we think there's something wrong with us if we have problems... ...But now you are letting go of disturbing thoughts... ...now and also when driving... ...and in doing so, you are also letting go of judgments and evaluations of your feelings... ...and this is why fear can also fade away... ...

You are preparing to do something that makes it even easier for you to let go of disturbing thoughts and self-judgments... ...You can already do this today... ...You simply let go of worrying thoughts and anticipatory fear by not judging them anymore... ...You let them be and at the same time focus on your new and helpful thought... ...Your new thought spreads, and the fear fades away... ...and with your thought, you actively approach driving... ...When getting in the car, you say... ...I now truly let go of all fear, and in doing so, I gain freedom and calmness when driving... ...and you immediately feel your body relaxing, which indeed becomes calmer with this thought... ...and then you know that you can actually drive... ...you can drive and feel good about it... ...You will approach this in your waking life... ...You get into the car with deliberate and focused thoughts... ...and you drive with conscious thoughts... ...with confidence... ...From now on, confidence and the feeling of freedom will accompany you when driving... ...From now on, true confidence and real freedom will accompany you when driving... ...

Driving is waiting for you... ...Driving in freedom and with real confidence is waiting for you in your waking life... ...You have initiated a clear change within yourself; you made it possible, and you set it up yourself... ...You have firmly imprinted a good and helpful thought into your subconscious today... ...your thought of easy driving... ...your thought that says... ...I now truly let go of all fear, and in doing so, I gain freedom and calmness when driving... ...and because you are now in such a stable trance, in a truly special trance, this thought will also become reality in your waking life... ...Maybe you're wondering what exactly is special about this trance... ...or you simply have a feeling for it and sense within yourself that this trance is indeed special... ...Your fearless driving will prove it to you... ...The feeling of freedom and your noticeable confidence while driving will show and prove it to you...

Hypnosis 2

You have an important goal... ...You want to drive a car again with ease... ...to feel good while doing it... ...just like before... ...Today, you want to let go of the fear and find new courage... ...You focus intently on this goal and fully concentrate on it... ...and that's why today, you are truly successful in overcoming fear and finding courage... ...You are successful today because you are completely focused on your goal of relaxed driving, truly completely focused... ...Your will is stronger than ever before; you want it today more than ever, so you are setting yourself up with all your strength and will to walk the path to relaxed driving today... ...Today, you are taking this step... ...Today, you are taking a more important and bigger step toward calmness and strength... ...and new courage... ...Today, you are even taking the most important step of all because today you are choosing a very special method, your trance... ...Today is your day of success... ...You are truly experiencing success today, more than you thought or expected... ...Today, you are reaching your goal of calm driving... ...of relaxed driving... ...Today... ...

First, you activate your inner strength and power because it helps you overcome fear... ...You can do this because you are fully focused on it... ...You have the power of success within you... ...It lies deep within you, and today you activate it... ...and then you can use it to overcome the fear of driving... ...and drive a car again with confidence... ...You can do it... ...Deep within you, there truly is this power of success because there have been several successes in your life... ...You know this, and now you are activating this power within you... ...Now... ...with your thoughts... ...Now... ...that's right... ...You really can do it... ...You are activating your power of success right now... ...You are overcoming your fear right now... ...You are also building new courage... ...It's happening... ...Your power of success is greater and stronger today than ever before... ...because in trance, you can use it more effectively than in your waking life... ...and now you are in trance... ...Now you are activating the power... ...Now you are using it... ...Now you are achieving your goal... ...

Deep within you... ...in your inner center, you now feel calm and balance... ...You can feel the calm and you know...

...In calmness lies strength... ...It unfolds now and makes driving seem harmless... ...because driving is harmless... ...You feel it within you... ...Driving is truly harmless... ...When you now think about driving, you remain completely calm and relaxed... ...because this thought is simple... ...as simple as driving without fear itself... ...as simple as relaxed driving itself... ...and this calm and relaxation... ...this serenity spreads and connects strongly with the idea of driving... ...with the idea of driving a car... ...If you want, relax even deeper... ...Let go even more and trust even more in the inner relaxation that you can now feel so well... ...and it becomes calmer within you... ...You go even deeper into trance and feel even more tired and comfortable... ...and the serenity becomes even more pronounced... ...and connects even more strongly with the idea of driving... ...with driving itself... ...Driving is completely normal for you... ...a routine event... ...Driving is completely normal for you... ...You remain calm when thinking about it again... ...Fear must now truly go away because it has long since become obsolete... ...has become useless... ...Serenity now completely replaces the fear... ...Serenity... ...Yes, serenity... ...

More and more, the former fear is now even replaced by anticipation... ...because you are already looking forward to driving a car again with ease... ...finally being able to act freely and move freely with the car... ...Anticipation now becomes stronger... ...Fear fades completely, and in its place now comes anticipation of driving... ...anticipation of driving a car... ...Anticipation becomes stronger than you thought... ...You can actually feel it when you listen deep within yourself... ...Fear thus fades completely, and in its place now truly and genuinely comes anticipation of driving... ...anticipation of driving a car... ...This is your new feeling... ...Anticipation, because there is indeed reason to look forward... ...You have shed the fear and focused on your successes... ...This is cause for anticipation because it allows you to drive again... ...You can do it... ...You really can do it... ...

You feel good and are now allowed to be proud of what you have achieved... ...You faced the fear and tackled it... ...You neutralized it and then replaced it with anticipation... ...Anticipation of driving... ...Anticipation of driving a car... ...You feel good, and you are proud to have achieved this... ...really achieved it, to have overcome the fear... ...This is a big step... ...a big step into freedom... ...You can be very proud of yourself and thank yourself for it... ...you may also praise yourself because it is you who has changed everything... ...It has always been you... ...These are just my words that you are hearing... ...But you are turning them into truth... ...your truth about relaxed driving... ...

Excellent, the most important step is behind you... ...Driving is now possible again... ...and what is possible, you will also put into practice in your daily life... ...You are successful... ...You are driving again and experiencing it as completely normal... ...It will be easier than you thought... ...and maybe you'll even be surprised at how well it goes and how relaxed you can be while doing it... ...You will experience day by day that it gets easier... ...With each time, it gets easier and more enjoyable to drive a car... ...Every drive becomes its own success... ...and you collect successes day after day... ...You can do it... ...You have already done it... ...You have truly already done it...

Hypnosis 3

You have come here today with a clear goal... ...You have often dealt with finding solutions to difficulties and problems... ...including solving the fear of driving... ...You've tried to do something about it so that you can drive more freely and calmly again... ...You've tried to let go of the fear because it could only hinder and bother you... ...It blocked you and restricted your freedom and didn't want to go away yet... ...But today will be different because today you don't even have to deal with it... ...Today, you can just let everything happen, and perhaps you will be surprised at how much faster the fear can fade away... ...So don't do anything now and don't try to help me... ...

There is one thing you can do, though... ...You can follow a simple mental image... ...You can imagine a very simple picture that I will present to you in a few moments... ...Then all you have to do is imagine it, and it's really simple... ...It happens automatically when I talk about it... ...The better you can focus solely on this image, the faster the fear will disappear... ...or more precisely: the faster you will be free again... ...free when driving... ...

You've experienced it like this... ...Just at the thought of driving, you felt fear... ...But from now on, this is how it should be... ...

Complete and lasting freedom from feelings of fear, trust, and calmness with every thought of driving.

... [Feel free to place your palm on the client's solar plexus while pronouncing the goal and then remove it again. This is not necessary, but it helps a lot because the goal is "anchored" this way. Of course, you can also incorporate energetic techniques into the hypnosis. Make sure not to repeat the goal.] ...

Now, focus your attention on your breath and feel how your breath flows in and out... ...in and out... ...[in the client's breathing rhythm]... ...in and out... ...in and out... ...and now continue to pay attention to the flow of your breath and imagine the light of a candle... ...Imagine the glow of the candle clearly... ...bright and clear... ...pleasantly warm and beautiful... ...Focus entirely on the image of the candlelight and let it grow with each inhale... ...with each inhale, the glow of the candle expands and grows... ...and with each exhale, the light of the candle becomes brighter... ...[in the client's breathing rhythm]... ...with each inhale, bigger and bigger... ...and with each exhale, brighter and brighter... ...with each inhale, bigger... ...And with each exhale, brighter... ...That's right... ...The glow of the candle is like a shining sun that expands... ...that lets its light grow larger and brighter... ...Only this image is important... ...only the image of the glowing candle, whose light changes... ...with each inhale, bigger... ...and with each exhale, brighter... ...The candlelight is now as big as a ball and continues to expand... ...a glowing ball that gets bigger and bigger... ...and surrounds your body more and more... ...In just a few breaths, your entire body will be completely enveloped by this light... ...just a few more breaths, and it will happen... ...Your body is completely surrounded by the candlelight, which shines like a sphere... ...You are at the center of this light, which continues to grow larger and larger... ...With each inhale, it expands further... ...until it envelops the entire building you are in and continues to grow larger... ...and with each exhale, brighter... ...The larger the light sphere becomes, the faster it also grows... ...and soon it reaches beyond the clouds... ...and encompasses the entire Earth, becoming the Earth's atmosphere... ...a shining atmosphere that reaches into infinity... ...a huge sphere of light surrounds the entire Earth... ...and at the center of the light sphere, you are breathing in and out... ...You are the center of the light... ...You are in this moment the center of the world... ...

... ... Continue breathing calmly and evenly... ...calmly and evenly... ...and imagine how the candlelight gets smaller with each breath... ...with each breath, it becomes a little smaller... ...and smaller... ...The light returns to the room where you are, bringing with it the full power of the universe... ...into the center where you are... ...The light becomes smaller and brings with it the power of the Earth... ...and finally, the entire power of the world gathers in the flame of the candle... ...and becomes your inner strength... ...

That's good... ...Everything important has been done... ...Everything is now harmonized and balanced... ...Harmony and balance within you... ...Now let your thoughts wander... ...No thought is important now... ...There is nothing more to do, nothing more to accomplish because everything is already done... ...Everything has already been completed... ...Let go of the image of the candle now, as it will remain within you as a feeling...

Hypnosis 4

Fear while driving has bothered you for a long time... ...You understand that you cannot change the past; no one can... ...This fear has paralyzed you, has constantly gotten in your way... ...You have realized that it was exaggerated, that it is time to feel free again... ...It is important to change your inner attitude... ...the deep inner attitude... ...In your mind, this happens quickly, but today it will also succeed in your feelings... ...Today, you can experience the feeling of inner freedom... ...experience it and solidify it... ...and then get back into a car with this feeling of freedom and start driving...

Deep inside, in your feelings, there is a special place... ...the place of clarity... ...At this place, there is only white, pure light... ...You are now standing at this place, seeing light all around you... ...Imagine it, and then you are there in your feelings as well... ...white light all around you... ...only white light everywhere... ...Imagine white light and the feeling of freedom... ...You are standing on a very stable glass floor... ...You can look infinitely deep through the floor... ...But even there, you only see pleasant, white light... ...You look up and see only light above you... ...It's everywhere... ...pleasant and warm... ...It surrounds you like a warming coat... ...and in front of you, there is a glass wall... ...You can look through it and see only light behind it as well... ...complete freedom at the place of clarity... ...white... ...pure... ...warm... ...free...

You look at the wall... ...Slowly, a script in thick black letters appears on the wall, becoming clearer and clearer... ...You can read the script... ...You can read it clearly... ...On the glass wall, at the place of clarity, it is written for you...

I let go of fear today because it has long since become obsolete. I feel free, and with a feeling of freedom, I can drive a car.

... [Read the affirmation slowly and a little louder than the previous text to highlight it. Then pause for a perceived 30 seconds before continuing to read.] ...

Take in these words and make them your own... ...Let their effect fully unfold and allow yourself to be calm and mindful... ...Calmness and mindfulness from you for yourself... ...Calmness and mindfulness from you for yourself... ...Let the effect of these words unfold... ...because everything you can allow and mindfully observe at the place of clarity deep within your feelings can fully unfold within you... ...always when it matches your desire and your goal... ...and you have this desire, this goal... ...Freedom within you... ...Freedom in the car... ...Letting go of fears... ...because deep inside, you know that you can... ...that you can let them go at the place of clarity... ...Maybe you can already feel the new freedom within you... ...or you will feel it even more strongly in a few moments because it is still unfolding... ...Yes, it will... ...It unfolds and becomes stronger until it becomes your stable fundamental attitude... ...your new attitude of inner freedom when driving... ...Freedom from fear because it has become obsolete... ...once served a function for you but is now no longer important... ...What matters now is the feeling of freedom when driving... ...your freedom when driving...

It's as if you are internally reading these words over and over again, saying them yourself... ...and letting them sink in even deeper...

I let go of fear today because it has long since become obsolete. I feel free, and with a feeling of freedom, I can drive a car.

… …Now, you can enjoy the calmness you are in… …excellent, how well you can feel calm with these words… …Calmness that shows you that you have indeed let go of the old fear now… …and can always let go again… …This is right and good… …this is very good… …At this moment, you are succeeding in absorbing the meaning of these words and turning them into a new and lasting fundamental attitude… …your attitude of freedom…

Excellent… …You have already done everything that needed to be done… …You have changed your fundamental attitude… …You have adopted a new and positive belief as an affirmation and anchored it deeply… …and as an affirmation, as the reinforcement of your correct belief… …your correct and constructive new attitude toward yourself, you can use this affirmation every day… …start every day with it… …and say it again and again…

I let go of fear today because it has long since become obsolete. I feel free, and with a feeling of freedom, I can drive a car.

… …This is how each new day begins at the place of clarity, and you can speak your freedom affirmation at the place of clarity every day… …Every day begins with your inner walk to the place of clarity… …With just one thought, you are there… …it's that simple… …You can read the words on the glass wall and, above all, feel them deep inside yourself… …and free yourself again and again… …every day…

Hypnosis 5

You have a goal... ...an important goal... ...You want to be able to drive a car again without fear and with a sense of security... ...You know the fear when getting into a car or driving... ...and there are certainly situations that are particularly difficult... ...But that is now over... ...because today, you can shift internally and regain freedom... ...learn again to drive freely and without constraint... ...In a trance, where you are right now, it is truly possible to find support in your subconscious... ...more help than in your waking life, where you have the problem of fear... ...Now, you are calm and relaxed, free from fear... ...and now you can even talk to your subconscious and decide what should happen... ...Your subconscious supports you because it hears and understands my words, which today become your own... ...because you say within yourself...

... ...I can and will drive a car again with a sense of security... ...because I know I could do it before... ...

... ...I can and will drive a car again with a sense of security... ...because I know I really want to deep down inside... ...

... ...I can and will drive a car again with a sense of security... ...because I know my subconscious is helping me with this... ...

... ...I can and will drive a car again with a sense of security... ...because I know my subconscious is following my goals today... ...

... ...So it shall be... ...So it shall and so it will be... ...

... ...I let go of fearful thoughts and focus on the thought that I am successful... ...and therefore, I can soon drive a car again calmly...

... ...I let go of fearful thoughts and focus on the thought that I am successful... ...and therefore, I can now calmly imagine driving again...

... ...I let go of fearful thoughts and focus on the thought that I am successful... ...and therefore, the thought of driving is pleasant for me again...

… …I let go of fearful thoughts and focus on the thought that I am successful… …and therefore, I am already looking forward to driving a car again calmly…

… …So it shall be… …So it shall and so it will be… …

… …The calmness my body feels now helps me stay calm in the car as well… …because what I can do now, I can do at any time…

… …The calmness my body feels now helps me stay calm in the car as well… …because I especially need a calm body when driving…

… …The calmness my body feels now helps me stay calm in the car as well… …because in this calmness, I can imagine everything and stay calm…

… …The calmness my body feels now helps me stay calm in the car as well… …because deep inside, this feeling of calmness is connected with the image of driving…

… …So it shall be… …So it shall and so it will be… …

… …I focus on my positive feelings and let them grow… …because positive feelings are always there…

… …I focus on my positive feelings and let them grow… …because fear is impossible with positive feelings…

… …I focus on my positive feelings and let them grow… …because this way I better recognize that I can have enough positive feelings when driving as well…

… …I focus on my positive feelings and let them grow… …because positive feelings help me strengthen my self-confidence…

… …So it shall be… …So it shall and so it will be… …

… …I actively and consciously approach driving… …because by confronting the car and driving, I overcome fear the fastest…

… …I actively and consciously approach driving… …because it is my firm intention to drive a car calmly again…

… …I actively and consciously approach driving… …because I also want to be able to drive alone again…

… …I actively and consciously approach driving… …because by doing so, I take control and power… …I am powerful… …I am truly powerful…

… …That's who I am… …That's really who I am… …[Now, stay silent for about 30 seconds]…

It works… …You have accepted all of this as your will deep inside… …Now, let all the words you have heard sink in deeply, and trust that they are your own and will be fulfilled just as you heard them… …Everything heard becomes internally spoken… …spoken by yourself… …and therefore, it truly succeeds that you can approach driving again… …and that you will soon be completely free and feel good when driving again… …You, fearless and confident in the car… …That's you… …That's really you…

Hypnosis 6

You have a goal... ...you want to be able to drive a car again... ...you want to be free from fear, completely natural, and with a calm feeling when driving your car... ...You know that deep inside, this fear lies, and that it can also be dissolved exactly there... ...only there... ...So today, it's about resolving this fear and finding another feeling just as deep inside... ...Rediscovering the confidence you once felt... ...and developing it anew... ...so that you can then drive a car again calmly and naturally... ...in all the situations that have caused you difficulties... ...To support this endeavor, you turn to an entity in which you can best believe... ...an entity you can truly believe in because you are convinced it will help you... ...and the words you hear from me become your inner words... ...You speak them with me because they reflect your will and your feeling...

Dear Subconscious / Dear Inner Helper / Dear Guardian Angel... ...Please help me overcome my fear... ...I know the strength for this lies within me, but I need support to find and develop it... ...Please help me see driving as normal again... ...by first letting go of the fear... ...because this loss of fear is a gain in freedom for me... ...a freedom that lies somewhere within me... ...as a feeling and as a memory because there was a time when I felt free and secure... ...in many situations... ...and also when driving... ...because driving was natural for me for a long time, and it can be again... ...with your help...

Dear Subconscious / Dear Inner Helper / Dear Guardian Angel... ...I thank you now for truly wanting to support me... ...because I know that this will help me better develop a new inner attitude and be able to drive again... ...I am sure that with your support and guidance, I can find the feeling of self-confidence within me again... ...I can find the confidence within me again and bring it to life... ...I, too, will do my part... ...I will do my best to find these helpful feelings... ...Dear Subconscious / Dear Inner Helper / Dear Guardian Angel... ...with your help, I am sure I will succeed... ...This way, I can feel and experience confidence again... ...and make it stronger... ...because with it, driving will become easier... ...and soon, it will become second nature...

Dear Subconscious / Dear Inner Helper / Dear Guardian Angel... ...I have understood that the fear mainly came about because too many burdens and experiences could not be adequately processed within me... ...I have also recognized that I am not to blame for this, but that it happened, and today I can even see it as a challenge... ...as a challenge that I accept and that I will also overcome... ...with your help and guidance, I am sure I will succeed... ...Dear Subconscious / Dear Inner Helper / Dear Guardian Angel... ...I trust that together we will succeed in dissolving the fear and replacing it with confidence... ...It is now time for new feelings... ...It is now time for confidence and security... ...Time to drive...

Dear Subconscious / Dear Inner Helper / Dear Guardian Angel... ...Please also help me to be patient... ...Patience that I may still need until I have fully succeeded in getting into a car with a good feeling and driving off... ...I know it will work, but I also know it may not work in this very second... ...But in a few days, the new confidence may have developed enough that I can drive calmly... ...So please help me to endure until then and accept myself in the meantime... ...Dear Subconscious / Dear Inner Helper / Dear Guardian Angel... ...Please also help me to be patient if it doesn't go as quickly as I wish... ...and to accept and tolerate myself even if I still feel some fear when driving...

...because even the rest of the fear will disappear... ...Dear Subconscious / Dear Inner Helper / Dear Guardian Angel... ...I thank you today for your support... ...Today and every day, because I know you are truly helping me...

Now, rest... ...Simply stay in your feeling and enjoy the calm and relaxation... ...because this is how the effect of the words unfolds best... ...Words you have heard... ...Words that a part of you has spoken internally... ...Words that reflect your desire and will... ...Trust in the support and guidance of your helping entity... ...and also in the support and guidance of your own inner strengths and experiences... ...Now, your confidence unfolds... ...Now, your confidence builds up again... ...stronger than ever before...

Hypnosis 7

You want to overcome the fear of driving and also the fear while driving... ...Indeed, these are two fears because you already think ahead with fear when it comes to the next drive, and then while driving, you experience a particular fear... ...today, you want to resolve both... ...you want to end the fear to be completely free again... ...You are particularly successful today in setting yourself up for an inner change... ...In the trance you are in, this is truly possible because, in trance, you are freer... ...Now, you are free from fear... ...even the thought of driving now keeps you calm... ...You can do it... ...you can stay calm when it comes to driving... ...and today we want to work together so that you can also do this in your waking life... ...on your next drive...

There was a time when you had no fear while driving... ...If you imagine you could just go back to that time and be free of fear again, it would be easy to end the fear... ...through a time travel... ...a journey into a fear-free time... ...But you live today, not in the past... ...But there is a better option that I choose with you today... ...an inner journey into the past, but this journey takes place in your feelings... ...because it is possible to revive past feelings and bring them into the present... ...Maybe you're wondering how that can work... ...or you've noticed that we're already on this journey, that you're already internally, in your feelings, on the way to the time before the fear... ...It's like a journey through your memories and experiences... ...and now that you know you're already on the way, images from the past can come up... ...Memories of the fear-free time... ...maybe you see yourself relaxed or even joyful in a car because you used to enjoy driving... ...Let these visual memories become clearer... ...You can remember clearly... ...For a long time, driving was completely okay for you... ...maybe even pleasant... ...Maybe you even really enjoyed driving... ...but certainly without fear... ...You drove completely naturally... ...it was easy... ...You are already internally in this time... ...You feel the lightness and calmness while driving... ...Lightness and calmness while driving...

Now immerse yourself in the images of that time and also in the light feeling of that time... ...You are experiencing this feeling now... ...here and today... ...A part of you is making this journey into the past, and a part of you is observing this special journey with me... ...and this part is happy for you and with you that you have found those past feelings again... ...They are becoming more and more clear... ...You feel the calmness of then now... ...You feel the calmness of then now... ...You clearly feel the ease with which you used to drive... ...Driving can feel this good... ...Driving can be this easy... ...You can get into a car this calmly... ...You can start driving this relaxed... ...and you can arrive at your destination this safely... ...because you have arrived at your destination a hundred times and more... ...You have arrived at your destination a hundred times and more completely safely... ...and you felt good about it... ...You remember... ...You remember clearly... ...Your body remembers and signals calmness and relaxation... ...Feel your body and feel how relaxed it is right now... ...Maybe you think your body is so relaxed because of the trance... ...and you are so calm inside because of the trance... ...But you think about driving and remain calm... ...much calmer than usual... ...The fear of driving is no longer there... ...The fear that has so often preceded you is no longer there... ...and with it, the fear while driving itself can also disappear... ...Focus completely on the calmness you can feel now... ...and with the next breaths, it can become even calmer within you... ...even calmer... ...and deep inside, this calmness and relaxation settle once more... ...You hold on to this calmness to bring it with you and use it every day... ...to stay calm every day when thinking about driving and then to drive a car again in a relaxed manner...

Your deep inner self reactivates this inner program of relaxed driving... ...because right now, this is happening... ...your old program of easy driving now becomes your new program of easy driving... ...your deep inner self holds on to easy driving... ...and with this easy driving program, your journey continues... ...You move into the future... ...You take an inner emotional journey into your future... ...You carry your easy driving program from the past into the future... ...and your confidence and self-assurance are active again... ...You can drive a car calmly again... ...Now... ...Now... ...You now look at images of the future... ...You imagine and see before your inner eye how it will be... ...You see yourself in the future in a car again without fear... ...You look calm... ...Driving is normal and easy...

What you could do before, you can also do in the near future... ...In the very near future, driving will be completely normal for you again... ...You see it, and you feel it... ...You know it, and you are sure... ...With this feeling, your journey continues... ...with the secure feeling that you have let go of the fear and are returning with old, new courage... ...With your new program full of confidence and strength, your journey continues into the present... ...You are coming step by step into the present and bringing your program of confidence when driving with you... ...You bring your program of self-assurance when arriving in the present with you... ...Fear is over, it's in the past... ...The present is confidence and courage... ...Confidence when driving... ...Courage when driving...

Hypnosis 8

Instructions for Implementation:

Ideomotor activity refers to the phenomenon where our body follows our feelings and thoughts with movements. In everyday life, this following is shown in body posture, muscle tension, and movement patterns of a person, which naturally change with mood and thoughts. In trance, ideomotor signals can be used to obtain information that the client cannot actively share. For example, the subconscious can answer questions with an agreed-upon finger signal. Of course, ideomotor responses can also be used suggestively, for example, with arm levitations and catalepsies. An ideomotor approach strengthens trust in hypnosis and one's ability to change, thus promoting therapy.

+++ End of Instructions +++

You have the goal of being able to drive a car again with a good feeling from now on... ...just getting in and driving off... ...and this can actually be achieved in cooperation with your subconscious… …because in hypnosis, in this deep relaxation where you are now, you can actually cooperate with your subconscious, and your subconscious can even show you that it is helping you… …Your subconscious will give you a signal and thereby confirm that you are both successful together and that you really can drive a car again without fear from now on… …I will help you, show you the way… …Maybe you're already wondering how exactly this works… …how your subconscious can show you that it has helped you and fulfilled your will… …So let's start, and then you will see…

Positive changes are always possible when it is successful to create a clear image of the goal and hold it… …and this clear image of the goal then unfolds… …imprints itself so firmly that it becomes a truth in our lives… …and you expect the truth of safe and relaxed driving to come to fruition… …So now it is especially important to have a clear image of this goal… …a vivid image of driving without fear and with ease… …So now, imagine what it looks like when you sit relaxed in the car and drive off… …Create a picture of it, as a fantasy, as a beautiful image… …First, imagine yourself sitting comfortably in the car while it's standing still…

...Adjust the seat so you can sit well and see everything well... ...Fasten your seatbelt... ...Consider and imagine how you can sit most comfortably and securely in the car... ...Then imagine yourself driving off calmly... ...maybe there's only your car on the road, making it even easier to drive now in your imagination... ...Imagine it now and feel that you are really calm while doing it... ...because now it's an image, a beautiful fantasy... ...so you stay calm... ...completely calm... ...You are in complete safety... ...You are truly in safety... ...You are driving relaxed in the car... ...The image imprints itself on you and becomes your new truth... ...Now, imagine it clearly, very clearly... ...and stay in this image... ...Keep driving... ...It's important that you stay in this feeling and that you stay in this image... ...The more you manage to keep this image now, the faster the fear fades and is completely replaced by calmness... ...You, relaxed while driving... ...You, completely relaxed while driving...

Stay entirely in this image... ...Imagine it like a movie playing out in front of you, completely under your control... ...because exactly this movie of relaxed driving is to become your truth, is to shape your everyday life again... ...because this is how you want to be again... ...this is how you want to drive again... ...this is how you want to drive a car again... ...Your deep inner self helps with this... ...The better you manage to maintain this image as an inner movie and see it before your inner eye, the better your deep inner self can turn it into truth... ...and as soon as your subconscious has done that, and it will do it, it will clearly move a finger on your right hand... ...as a sign that you can really hold this inner image and that it will become truth... ...Your subconscious will show you when it is ready, when it has taken this on for you... ...As soon as the fear is gone and calmness is connected with driving, your subconscious will move a finger on your right hand... ...Your subconscious will do it, it will move a finger clearly and tell you that you can drive a car calmly... ...as soon as you are awake again... ...Your subconscious will move a finger, and it does not lie... ...As soon as a finger on your right hand moves clearly, this is the commitment from your subconscious that you can drive a car calmly again... ...It keeps its commitment...

[Please try to be patient until a finger clearly moves. Ideomotor signals are reliable signs, similar to kinesiology muscle tests. Here, we are working with a mix of suggestive prompting and ideomotor communication. If you repeatedly say... Your hand closes into a fist... it has a suggestive effect, and the ideomotor response follows. By associating this with fearlessness, a connection is made in the unconscious. The subconscious thus confirms the relaxed driving at the same time. If it could not end the fear, it would not make sense to move a signal finger. So, if the closing occurs only due to suggestion, it is still proof of effectiveness for the conscious mind since it was "agreed upon." If the mind is convinced, the goal is almost reached].

Your subconscious has confirmed the image of fear-free and relaxed driving, and therefore, it will be so... ...Your fingers are now becoming fully mobile again, and you have full control over your hand... ...Your subconscious is handing back full control of your right hand to you, and it relaxes... ...Simply move the fingers of your right hand or even both hands and feel that they are loose and under your control...

[Always make sure that the client has regained conscious and active control over their hands and fingers and can move them. Encourage them to actively try. If it doesn't work, help with more suggestions... Your hands and fingers are totally relaxed, completely loose. Your hands and fingers are completely loose... You can move them...]

Your subconscious has worked with you to resolve the fear and build a sense of security... ...You have helped with your vivid imagination, and your subconscious with anchoring the image and with the signal finger as confirmation that you can drive a car without fear from now on... ...So you can be sure that you will really succeed...

Hypnosis 9

Instructions for Implementation:

In this hypnosis, a self-hypnosis trigger is trained. A self-hypnosis trigger is a signal that initiates the state of trance. With its help, even an inexperienced client can continue working with self-hypnosis at home. Of course, they can work "only" with simple suggestions that they can easily remember and that we should prepare, or with simple visualizations. Triggered self-hypnosis is a very good tool to give the client a task to take with them and to promote therapy. This way, the time between sessions in practice is not without therapy, but it is continued at home.

A completely self-directed self-hypnosis, without a trigger, is also easy to learn but requires a lot of time and practice. Setting up the trigger is a fairly simple task and naturally relieves the client, whom I do not want to burden with training self-directed self-hypnosis. Despite all the skeptics, I also claim here that it is really not a problem to teach a client simple trigger self-hypnosis. It is no more dangerous than meditation, autogenic training, or yoga. You can survive all of these at home unscathed. I have experienced numerous patients in my practice who not only handled self-hypnosis well but also enjoyed it. And if a patient enjoys self-hypnosis, no matter how simple the suggestion may seem, then that is a very good support for compliance.

Discuss the process once before hypnosis and give the client a brief, bullet-point list of the steps of self-hypnosis so they have a small guide.

+++ End of Instructions +++

I will now practice self-hypnosis with you because self-hypnosis can really help you lose your fear in the car... ...to let go of the fear while driving... ...and drive a car again naturally... ...You can do self-hypnosis at any time... ...but it's best to do it early in the morning or just before bed... ...You can repeat it as often as you want... ...Each repetition helps you lose fear faster and drive a car without constraint again... ...Now, focus your attention on the feeling of relaxation, on the state of trance that you are in at this moment... ...

It feels calm and relaxed... ...really calm and relaxed and at the same time completely normal, completely natural... ...You can create and actively use this state yourself... ...It's really easy, and I will show you today how it's done... ...Now, feel the calm and relaxation clearly... ...Feel how good it feels to be so relaxed... ...in trance and still hearing everything around you...

You can go into trance at any time... ...even at home... ...For this, you use a little trick... ...You close your eyes several times in a row and whisper... ...I, in trance... ...With open eyes, you whisper... ...I... ...and when closing your eyes, you then quietly say... ...in trance... ...and you repeat this until you clearly feel your eyes getting tired... ...and this happens very quickly because you are learning it now... ...

So, make yourself comfortable at home, as comfortable as possible... ...Then start with open eyes and whisper... ...I... ...Then slowly close your eyes and whisper... ...in trance... ...and immediately open your eyes again... ...Then repeat this until you feel tiredness in your eyes... ...Then you can keep them closed and relax... ...Then you feel that your eyes relax again...

Just like here, you can also deepen the trance to relax even better... ...It's simple again... ...Whisper ten times... ...I in trance even deeper... ...and count to ten... ...It goes like this... ...I, in trance once deeper... ...I, in trance twice deeper... ...I, in trance three times deeper... ... ...and so on... ...until you finally reach ten and whisper... ...I, in trance ten times deeper... ...and with this whispering and counting, you go into a really pleasant trance... ...A part of you remains awake enough to keep whispering and steer your self-hypnosis... ...Everything is in order and goes easily...

[For deepening and main part, I recommend counting with the suggestions... once... twice, etc. This has the advantage that the client is not distracted by the question of how often they have now repeated the suggestion. It doesn't really matter if it's ten repetitions, but in trance, they can more easily keep track this way. You can, of course, speak all ten repetitions. After all, in this hypnosis, you are also working suggestively. So it is not just a self-hypnosis training but also hypnosis.]

Then you move on to the main part, which is really important for your self-hypnosis... ...and in this part, you use a special self-suggestion... ...You whisper it ten times again...

...Ten times you say... ...I can and will drive calmly... ...Remember, always count... ...So say... ...I can and will drive calmly once... ...I can and will drive calmly twice... ...I can and will drive calmly three times... ...and finally... ...I can and will drive calmly ten times... ...and then you may simply enjoy the calmness of the trance and don't have to do anything more... ...You may simply enjoy the calmness afterward...

You then need to wake yourself up, and that's also easy... ...It's easy because you're learning it now, in trance because your subconscious is learning for you... ...Imagine a cold wind blowing, and it's really cold... ...Then say loudly and clearly... ...Time to wake up... ...and quickly and loudly count to three and open your eyes... ...It's really easy, so once again... ...To wake yourself up, imagine a freezing cold wind blowing into your face... ...and then say loudly and clearly... ...Time to wake up – one – two – three... ...and then you are really awake and can open your eyes... ...It's really that simple...

You have understood and internalized how it works... ...You can now do self-hypnosis and continue working on driving again... ...Your subconscious has learned for you to go into trance immediately, and you know how to proceed... ...The closing and opening of the eyes take you into trance, which you deepen with the words I, in trance even deeper... ...Then comes your suggestion... I can and will drive calmly... and at the end, imagine freezing cold wind and say... Time to wake up – one – two – three...

Hypnosis 10

You are getting ready for a very special journey... ...a journey that takes place deep in your thoughts and feelings... ...somewhere in the creativity of your imagination... ...But imagination and reality are the same if you can allow it... ...if you allow your imagination to become the new truth in your life... ...So you are preparing to find a new truth deep within your imagination and creativity... ...in a land where anything you wish and dream of is possible... ...in a land that lies deep within yourself... ...the land of dreams... ...with just one breath, you reach it... ...You can take this breath now because the time has come to go there and start anew... ...You are going to the land of dreams...

You have experienced a lot in your life... ...There were also difficult times and, above all, times when you felt you were losing yourself... ...because you had no time for your own feelings... ...You had so much to take care of that there was no time... ...and so, over time, too many unseen feelings and emotions accumulated within you... ...It was like an overpressure that suddenly began to discharge as fear...

...You often asked yourself why you actually had this fear while driving, couldn't really explain it... ...These are the feelings of the past that are finding their way... ...You think about how you would like to change the past... ...some things you have experienced, you would like to undo, maybe even some of what you once said or did... ...But all that is not possible... ...The past is over, and therefore it cannot be changed anymore, and there can be no compensation... ...whatever was once done to you... ...whatever was denied to you... ...It cannot be undone because that would only be possible if the past could actually be changed... ...Any compensation or comfort you could receive would not undo anything... ...So you are here today to let go, to let go of the desire for compensation... ...You don't have to forgive anything; that remains solely your own decision... ...the land of dreams leaves it to you whether and what or whom you will ever forgive... ...but that's not the point...

... ...You are standing at a crossroads in the land of dreams... ...You hear the sound of engines and see cars approaching you... ...They are coming from all sides of the crossroads, but you stand still... ...The cars slow down and finally stop... ...People get out and come to you... ...They are people you know from your life... ...Some of them you meet often in your present... ...others you may have met in the past and see them again today... ...The images of the people who should be here today appear on their own... ...These are the people who have contributed to your fear... ...many of them didn't even know that your fear would arise... ...but everyone who comes into our lives contributes to what we are and how we think and feel... ...just as we contribute to their development and feelings... ...More and more cars are coming to the crossroads, and more and more people are getting out... ...you probably didn't expect some of them, and maybe you don't even know some of them because you don't consciously notice every person who comes into your life... ...You discover some people who remind you most of your own life story because they played an important role in it... ...some have helped you a lot, others have made your life harder... ...But you are here to say goodbye to them... ...to say goodbye to everything that was in the past... ...You can now say what you want to say... ...in the world of your imagination, in the land of dreams, you can now say what you have always wanted to say... ...whatever it may be... ...You don't have to be friendly and not polite either... ...just follow your feelings… …Speak inwardly calmly what you want to say… …I will give you time now and get back to you in a minute to move on with you…

… … [Now, please stay silent for about a minute. Then continue reading.] …

… …You hear the sound of engines and see a light blue, new car coming to the crossroads… …a big, fast car, and at the wheel is a child who looks like you did as a child… …You yourself are this child, more precisely, a part of you is this child… …Here in the land of dreams, it is your inner child who drives the car safely… …It comes to pick you up… …The car stops, and you get in… …The people stay at the crossroads, you leave them behind… …The child accelerates and drives faster and faster… …You look around and see the people at the crossroads slowly dissolving into white mist… …You enjoy the ride and feel really good… …You feel free and sense that it was the burdens of the old times that led to this fear… …Fear that actually had nothing to do with driving… …It just discharged there… …But today you have cleared it up… …you have said what has remained unsaid so far… …you have freed yourself from the inner pressure… …and that's why you can enjoy the ride… …You feel liberated and enjoy the ride... ...a really fast ride, and you trust the child who is driving the car... ...You trust your inner child... ...Far away, the child stops the car, and you get out...

You breathe in deeply and look up at the light blue sky... ...The sky looks huge and wide... ...there are no clouds... ...only the free, beautiful sky... ...and deep inside, you feel just as free and vast as the sky... ...free and vast... ...Then you think about how you can experience the same feeling in your waking life because everything that is possible here is also possible there... ...because the land of dreams is more than imagination... ...It is a truth... ...a truth within you... ...the truth of your feelings... ...But where exactly is this land?... ...The land of dreams lies deep within you... ...it has always been there... ...I am just telling you about it...

Distribution, publication, and copying in any form are prohibited and subject to damages.

All Titles in the Series

Volume 1: Smoking Cessation
Volume 2: Anxiety and Restlessness
Volume 3: Burnout
Volume 4: Reducing Overweight
Volume 5: Coping with the Past
Volume 6: Suicidal Thoughts and Attempts
Volume 7: Psycho-Oncology
Volume 8: Obsessions and Tics
Volume 9: Self-Confidence and Decision-Making
Volume 10: Grief Work
Volume 11: Psychosomatics
Volume 12: Chronic Pain
Volume 13: Depressive Thoughts
Volume 14: Panic Attacks
Volume 15: Domestic Violence, Victim Support
Volume 16: Post-Traumatic Stress
Volume 17: Exam Anxiety and Stage Fright
Volume 18: Anti-Violence Training, Offender Support
Volume 19: Addiction Tendencies
Volume 20: Social Phobia and Fear of Contact
Volume 21: Nail Biting
Volume 22: Self-Awareness and Self-Love
Volume 23: Teeth Grinding and Night Clenching
Volume 24: Feelings of Guilt
Volume 25: Fear in Crowds
Volume 26: Fear of Flying, Aviophobia
Volume 27: Fear in Enclosed Spaces, Claustrophobia
Volume 28: Tinnitus, Ear Noises
Volume 29: Fear of Heights
Volume 30: Neurodermatitis

Copying, publishing, and sharing with third parties are only permitted with the written consent of the author. Please observe the notes on copyright and usage.

Volume 31: Finding Inner Balance
Volume 32: Overcoming Loneliness
Volume 33: Fear of Illness, Hypochondria
Volume 34: Anticipatory Anxiety, Fear of Fear
Volume 35: Jealousy in Relationships
Volume 36: Driving Anxiety
Volume 37: New Start after Separation
Volume 38: Fear of Injections
Volume 39: Heart Anxiety Neurosis
Volume 40: Overcoming Resentment and Anger
Volume 41: Resolving Blockages and Positive Thinking
Volume 42: Stress Reduction, Stress Management
Volume 43: Body Relaxation
Volume 44: Deep Relaxation
Volume 45: Fear of the Dark
Volume 46: Falling Asleep and Staying Asleep
Volume 47: Compulsive Buying
Volume 48: Restless Legs Syndrome
Volume 49: Bulimia
Volume 50: Anorexia
Volume 51: Overcoming Nightmares
Volume 52: Imagined Deformity
Volume 53: Overcoming Distrust, Finding Trust
Volume 54: Processing Failures
Volume 55: Humiliation, Emotional Hurt
Volume 56: Distressing Compassion, Vicarious Suffering
Volume 57: Self-Forgiveness
Volume 58: Self-Awareness, Self-Confidence
Volume 59: Saying No
Volume 60: Assertiveness
Volume 61: Setting Boundaries and Self-Assertion
Volume 62: Decision-Making Ability

- Volume 63: Success Orientation
- Volume 64: Ruminating, Circular Thinking
- Volume 65: Accepting Pregnancy
- Volume 66: Birth Preparation
- Volume 67: Spiritual Opening
- Volume 68: Joy of Life and Inner Lightness
- Volume 69: Patience and Inner Peace
- Volume 70: Fibromyalgia and Rheumatism
- Volume 71: Irritable Bowel Syndrome, Crohn's Disease
- Volume 72: Fear of Nausea, Emetophobia
- Volume 73: Stuttering and Cluttering, Speech Flow Disorders
- Volume 74: Concentration and Knowledge Anchoring
- Volume 75: Vitality and Spontaneity
- Volume 76: Searching for Meaning and Finding Goals
- Volume 77: Life Crises, Life Events
- Volume 78: Workaholism, Goal Obsession
- Volume 79: Helper Syndrome, Helpless Helpers
- Volume 80: Medication Abuse
- Volume 81: Gambling Addiction
- Volume 82: Internet Addiction, Smartphone Addiction
- Volume 83: Hoarding Disorder, Compulsive Collecting
- Volume 84: Conspiracy Thoughts, Overvalued Ideas
- Volume 85: Fear of Operations and Treatments
- Volume 86: Fear of Aging
- Volume 87: Travel Anxiety
- Volume 88: Anxiety When Urinating, Paruresis
- Volume 89: Fear of Intimacy and Togetherness
- Volume 90: Fear of Blushing
- Volume 91: Coming Out in Homosexuality
- Volume 92: Charisma Training
- Volume 93: Migraines and Chronic Headaches
- Volume 94: Overcoming Allergies, Bronchial Asthma

Volume 95: Normalizing Blood Pressure
Volume 96: Compulsive Perfectionism
Volume 97: Sports Hypnosis, Motivation
Volume 98: Sports Hypnosis, Performance Enhancement
Volume 99: Determination and Focus
Volume 100: Encountering the Inner Child
Volume 101: Cravings, Binge Eating
Volume 102: Stimulating Metabolism
Volume 103: Bipolar Mood Swings
Volume 104: Borderline, Identity Crises
Volume 105: Hypomania, Euphoria, Mania
Volume 106: Restlessness, Agitation
Volume 107: Nervous Breakdown
Volume 108: Adjustment Disorders
Volume 109: Self-Alienation, Depersonalization
Volume 110: Ending Self-Pity
Volume 111: Primary Gain of Illness
Volume 112: Secondary Gain of Illness
Volume 113: Bullying, Victim Support
Volume 114: Letting Go of Envy and Jealousy
Volume 115: Fear of Spiders, Arachnophobia
Volume 116: Fear of Dogs or Cats
Volume 117: Fear of Strangers, Xenophobia
Volume 118: Excessive Worries, Generalized Anxiety
Volume 119: Strengthening Sense of Responsibility
Volume 120: Unrequited Love, Heartache
Volume 121: Work-Life Balance
Volume 122: Letting Go of Unattainable Goals
Volume 123: Allowing and Accepting Help
Volume 124: Letting Go of Adult Children
Volume 125: Tourette Syndrome
Volume 126: Life Changes and New Starts

Volume 127: Accepting Life in a Wheelchair
Volume 128: Understanding and Overcoming Homesickness
Volume 129: Understanding and Overcoming Wanderlust
Volume 130: Dizziness, Meniere's Disease
Volume 131: Overcoming Aggression
Volume 132: Cutting and Self-Harm
Volume 133: Hair Pulling, Trichotillomania
Volume 134: Postpartum Depression
Volume 135: For Relatives of Dementia Patients
Volume 136: Self-Harm, Artificial Disorders
Volume 137: Activating Self-Healing Powers
Volume 138: Preventing Depression Relapse
Volume 139: Reactive Psychoses, Follow-Up
Volume 140: Obsessive Thoughts and Impulses
Volume 141: Compulsive Checking
Volume 142: Compulsive Counting, Symmetry Obsession
Volume 143: Compulsive Washing, Cleanliness Obsession
Volume 144: Compulsive Questioning
Volume 145: Dissociative Paralysis
Volume 146: Phantom Pain
Volume 147: Overcoming Complaining
Volume 148: Hay Fever, Pollen Allergy
Volume 149: Sexual Abuse, Victim Support
Volume 150: Standing Strong Against Sexism, #metoo
Volume 151: Binge Eating
Volume 152: Overcoming Thoughts of Revenge
Volume 153: Detachment from the Aggressor, Stockholm Syndrome
Volume 154: Courage to Separate
Volume 155: Chronic Fatigue, Exhaustion
Volume 156: Fear of the Future, Existential Anxiety
Volume 157: Excessive Worry About Children
Volume 158: Fear of Failure

Volume 159: Ending Distrust and Control
Volume 160: Dejection, Dysphoria
Volume 161: Boreout, Chronic Boredom
Volume 162: Bipolar Disorders, Relapse Prevention
Volume 163: Mania, Relapse Prevention
Volume 164: Nihilism, Feelings of Worthlessness
Volume 165: Thumb Sucking
Volume 166: Being Brave
Volume 167: Being Proud
Volume 168: Overcoming Shyness
Volume 169: Being Able to Delegate Responsibility
Volume 170: Being Able to Show Emotions
Volume 171: Letting Go of Guilt, Victim Support
Volume 172: Processing Guilt, Offender Support
Volume 173: Mood Swings, Cyclothymia
Volume 174: Lack of Drive, Vital Sadness
Volume 175: Hearing Voices with Reality Reference
Volume 176: Confident Communication
Volume 177: Standing Up for Oneself
Volume 178: Taking New Paths
Volume 179: Confident Job Application
Volume 180: No Longer Being Taken Advantage Of
Volume 181: End of Submissiveness
Volume 182: Depressive Numbness
Volume 183: Mood Drops, Affective Incontinence
Volume 184: Mood Instability
Volume 185: Somatoform Disorders
Volume 186: Stomach Ulcer, Psychosomatic
Volume 187: Accepting Amputation
Volume 188: Overcoming and Letting Go of Hatred
Volume 189: Ending Accusations
Volume 190: Allowing Tears, Being Able to Cry

Volume 191: Finding and Sorting Repressed Feelings
Volume 192: Somatoform Pain
Volume 193: Living Autonomously
Volume 194: Anhedonia, Joylessness
Volume 195: Persistent Sadness
Volume 196: Obesity, Food Addiction
Volume 197: Parents of Abused Children
Volume 198: Letting Go and Letting Be
Volume 199: Childhood Sexual Abuse
Volume 200: Fear of Loss

www.ingramcontent.com/pod-product-compliance
Lightning Source LLC
Chambersburg PA
CBHW030503220526
45464CB00006B/2631